# My Vegetable
# ADVENTURES

A Journal for Food Discovery and
Exploration Using Your 5 Senses

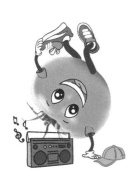 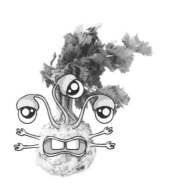 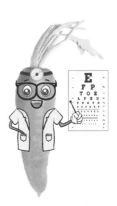

This journal be.'

D12221177

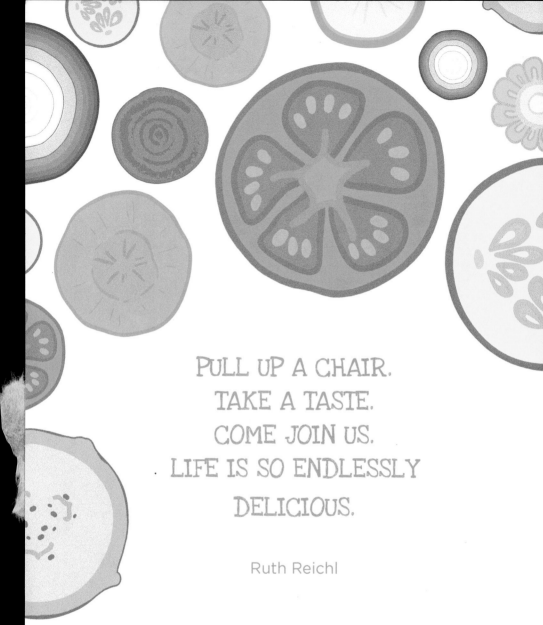

PULL UP A CHAIR.
TAKE A TASTE.
COME JOIN US.
. LIFE IS SO ENDLESSLY
DELICIOUS.

Ruth Reichl

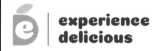

**experience
delicious**

Experience Delicious LLC

Copyright 2019 Experience Delicious, LLC.
ISBN: 978-1-947001-16-9
www.experiencedeliciousnow.com

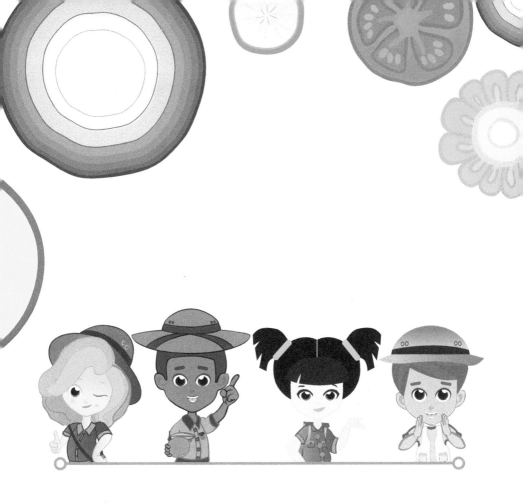

# Welcome Food Explorer!

It's time to experiment with veggies using your five senses!
Conduct your own taste-tests with new vegetables or old favorites
prepared in different ways. Try different varieties of the same
vegetable side by side. Learn how to use descriptive words while
discovering flavors and textures. Get ready to learn more about
YOUR veggie preference

This journal is your personal vegetable ex            designed
to track your adventures with veggies a              for you
to write and talk about what you like a              ut them.

Don't forget to include your parents, caregivers, and friends
on your search for delicious and ask for help when needed!
Now put on your Food Explorer hat, pick a vegetable to try, grab
your crayons or colored pencils, and dig in!

# Let's start by drawing your favorite veggie!

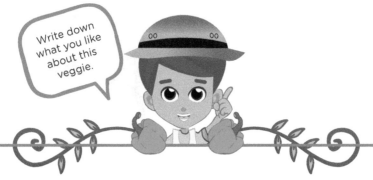

Write down what you like about this veggie.

# Next, draw your
# least favorite veggie.

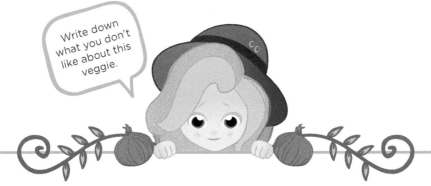

Write down what you don't like about this veggie.

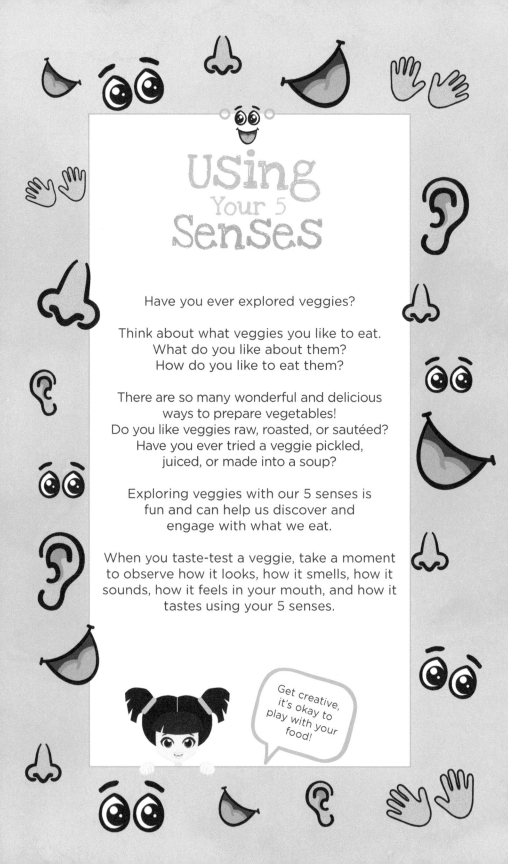

# USing
### Your 5
# SenSes

Have you ever explored veggies?

Think about what veggies you like to eat.
What do you like about them?
How do you like to eat them?

There are so many wonderful and delicious
ways to prepare vegetables!
Do you like veggies raw, roasted, or sautéed?
Have you ever tried a veggie pickled,
juiced, or made into a soup?

Exploring veggies with our 5 senses is
fun and can help us discover and
engage with what we eat.

When you taste-test a veggie, take a moment
to observe how it looks, how it smells, how it
sounds, how it feels in your mouth, and how it
tastes using your 5 senses.

Get creative,
it's okay to
play with your
food!

# 5 Senses

Can you describe a vegetable? Each preparation method can change the experience. We can use our 5 senses to discover things we never knew we liked about a food!

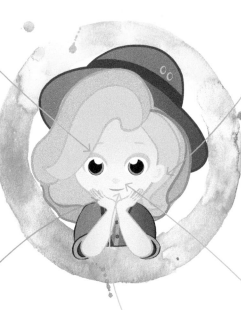

## See

Take a closer look at the veggie. What colors and textures do you SEE? Does it remind you of anything?

## Hear

What sound do you HEAR when you run your fingers over the skin? Is it silent or does it make a sound? Now take a bite. Did you HEAR anything? Keep chewing. Are there any sounds? Is each bite a loud crunch or a quiet chew?

## Feel

How does the skin FEEL in your hands? Is the texture rough, smooth, or silky? What about when you peel the skin? What does the texture FEEL like in your hands or when you take a bite? Is it firm, sticky, or mushy? Is each bite soft and tender? Try it raw or prepared!

## Taste

How does it TASTE? What is the flavor like? Can you describe it? Is it sweet or sour? Does it have a flavor at all? Does it TASTE different when it is raw than when it is prepared another way? Which do you like better and why?

## Smell

Have you ever sniffed your veggies? That might sound silly, but SMELLING food is a big part of tasting! Hold a piece of a veggie up to your nose and take a good whiff. What does it SMELL like? Does it SMELL earthy, herbal, or pungent? Does it have a scent at all?

# 100 Descriptive Words

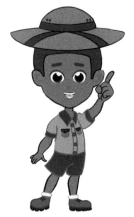

Descriptive words help us identify unique qualities about foods and explain what we like or dislike about them.

When you sit down for a meal or snack, take a moment to think about how it looks, how it smells, how it sounds, how it feels in your mouth, and how it tastes using your 5 senses. It's like your very own experiment every time you eat!

When a food feels, looks, smells, or tastes similar to another food you can say it is "like" another food or add a "y" at the end of the word. Such as butter-like, celery-like, or honey-like and citrusy, lemony, or watery.

| WORD | DESCRIPTION | SENSE(S) |
|---|---|---|
| Acidic | bitter, sharp, sour | Taste |
| Ambrosial | delicious, fragrant, sweet | Smell · Taste |
| Anise | herbal smell, sweet, tastes similar to licorice | Smell · Taste |
| Aroma; Aromatic | scent, smell, odor | Smell |
| Astringent | mouth-puckering, sharp | Taste |
| Bitter | acidic, harsh, sharp, sour | Taste |
| Bland | flavorless, mild | Taste |
| Bright | acidic, sharp, tart, giving out or reflecting light, shiny appearance | See · Taste |
| Buttery | creamy, rich, smooth, velvety, feels similar to butter | Feel · Taste |
| Chewy | leathery, sticky, tough | Feel |
| Citrusy | looks, smells, or tastes similar to a citrus fruit such as lemons, oranges, or grapefruit | See · Smell · Taste |
| Complex | multiple aromas, flavors, or textures | Feel · Smell · Taste |
| Creamy | smooth, velvety | Feel |
| Crisp(y) | crunchy, firm, snappy | Feel · Hear |
| Crumbly | breaks into pieces under pressure, brittle, crisp | Feel · See |
| Crunchy | brittle, crisp, loud | Feel · Hear |
| Delicate | fine texture, tender, light or subtle taste | Feel · Taste |
| Dense | compact, heavy, thick | Feel |
| Distinctive | unlike other textures or flavors, unique qualities | Feel · Taste |
| Dry | free of liquid or moisture | Feel · See · Taste |
| Dull | having little color, smell, or taste | See · Smell · Taste |
| Earthy | feels, smell, or tastes similar to soil | Feel · Smell · Taste |
| Exotic | different, unusual, unfamiliar | See · Taste |

| WORD | DESCRIPTION | SENSE(S) |
|---|---|---|
| Fibrous | stringy, thick, tough | Feel |
| Firm | hard, solid, stiff | Feel |
| Flavorful | having a lot of flavor | Taste |
| Flesh(y) | pulpy, soft, thick | Feel |
| Floral; Flowery | smell or taste similar to a flower | Smell · Taste |
| Fluffy | airy, light | Feel · See · Taste |
| Fragrant | sweet smell or scent, perfumed | Smell |
| Fresh | new, peak of ripeness, unspoiled | Feel · See · Smell · Taste |
| Fruity | varies and can mean citrusy, sweet, or tangy | Taste · Smell |
| Fuzzy | fibrous, furry, or hairy coating | Feel · See |
| Glossy | glazed, polished, shiny | See |
| Glutinous | gluey, starchy, sticky | Feel · See · Taste |
| Grainy | coarse, granular, gritty | Feel · See |
| Grassy | smell, taste, or feel similar to grass | Feel · Smell · Taste |
| Gritty | coarse, grainy, granular, rough | Feel · See · Taste |
| Hard | firm, solid | Feel |
| Hearty | large, filling, substantial, tough | Feel · See · Taste |
| Herbal | smell or taste similar to an herb | Smell · Taste |
| Honeyed | feels, looks, smells, or tastes similar to honey | Feel · See · Smell · Taste |
| Juicy | full of juice or liquid, succulent | Feel · Hear · See |
| Knobby | lumpy surface, rounded | See |
| Light | contains air, does not make you feel full quickly, lacks a strong color, smell or taste | Feel · See · Smell · Taste |
| Limp | soft, lifeless, un-firm | Feel · See |
| Mealy | crumbly, dry, grainy | Feel · See |
| Meaty | dense, thick, taste or texture similar to meat | Feel · Taste |
| Mild | bland, free of a strong smell or taste | Smell · Taste |
| Moist | slightly damp or wet | Feel · See |
| Mushy | may feel spoiled, soft, wet | Feel |
| Mustardy | smells or tastes similar to mustard | Smell · Taste |
| Musty | bad odor, moldy, stale | Smell · Taste |
| Nutty | tastes similar to nuts | Taste |
| Odor | aroma, musk, scent | Smell |
| Peppery | hot, pungent, spicy, smells or tastes similar to pepper | Smell · Taste |
| Plump | fleshy, full, round | Feel · See |
| Pulpy | fibrous, fleshy, soft | Feel · See |
| Pungent | bitter, hot, peppery, sharp, powerful smell or taste | Smell · Taste |
| Refreshing | cool, fresh, or different | Feel · Smell · Taste |
| Rich | creamy, dense, fatty, full-flavored, heavy, strong and pleasant smell or taste | Feel · Taste · Smell |
| Rotten | bad, moldy, spoiled | Taste · See · Smell |
| Rough | bumpy, textured, uneven surface | Taste · See · Feel |
| Rubbery | elastic, flexible, tough, similar to rubber | Feel · See |

| WORD | DESCRIPTION | SENSE(S) |
|---|---|---|
| Salty | tasting or containing salt | Taste |
| Savory | delicious smell or taste, having a salty or spicy quality without sweetness, well-seasoned | Taste · Smell |
| Seeded | having seeds | Feel · Hear · See |
| Sharp | distinct, powerful smell or taste, pungent | Taste · Smell |
| Shrivel | shrink, wither, wrinkle | Feel · See |
| Silky | glossy, smooth, soft, similar to silk | Feel · See |
| Slimy | gooey, slippery, wet, similar to slime | Feel · See |
| Smoky | smell or taste similar to smoke from a wood grill | Smell · Taste |
| Smooth | even, flat, uniform consistency | Feel · See |
| Soft | smooth, easy to press | Feel · See |
| Sour | acidic, bitter, tart, similar to lemon or vinegar | Feel · Smell · Taste |
| Spicy | aromatic, hot, peppery, pungent, strongly flavored | Smell · Taste |
| Spongy | airy, light, soft, feels similar to a sponge | Feel · See |
| Squeaky | high pitched sound | Hear |
| Stale | dry, old, musty, change in texture or appearance | Smell · Taste |
| Starchy | feel or taste similar to other high starch foods such as potatoes or rice | Feel · Taste |
| Sticky | glue-like, syrupy, tacky, viscous | Feel · See |
| Stinky | unpleasant smell | Smell |
| Stringy | fibrous, tough, similar to string-like pieces | Feel · See |
| Subtle | delicate, faint, light | Smell · Taste |
| Sugary | sweet, honeyed, similar to sugar | Feel · See · Smell · Taste |
| Sweet | smell or taste similar to sugar or honey | Smell · Taste |
| Sweet-Sour | both sweet and sour | Feel · Smell · Taste |
| Sweet-Tart | both sweet and tart | Feel · Smell · Taste |
| Tangy | aromatic, flavorful, sharp, strong | Smell · Taste |
| Tart | acidic, sharp, sour | Feel · Taste |
| Tender | delicate, soft | Feel |
| Tough | dense, fibrous, hard | Feel |
| Umami | meaty taste, one of the basic taste sensations along with bitter, salty, sour, and sweet | Taste |
| Velvety | delicate, smooth, soft | Feel |
| Watery | feels, looks, or tastes similar to water | Feel · See · Taste |
| Waxy | shiny, sticky, similar feel and look to wax | Feel · See |
| Woody | fibrous, feels, looks, or smells similar to wood | Feel · Smell · Taste |
| Wrinkly | bumps, creases, or folds on a surface | See |
| Zesty | pungent, seasoned, sharp, spicy, tart | Smell · Taste |
| Zippy | fresh, invigorating | Taste |

# Let's practice!

## Use 5 words to describe this veggie.

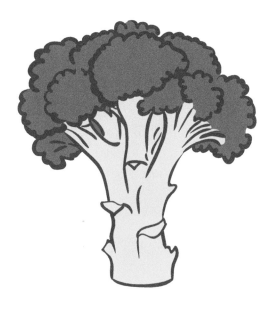

_____

_____

_____

_____

_____

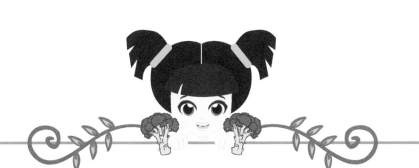

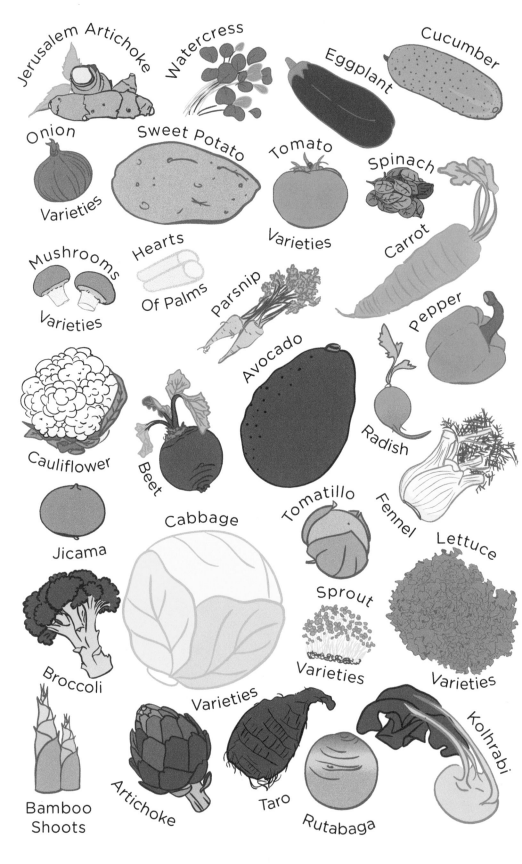

Jerusalem Artichoke

Watercress

Eggplant

Cucumber

Onion
Varieties

Sweet Potato

Tomato
Varieties

Spinach

Carrot

Mushrooms
Varieties

Hearts
Of Palms

Parsnip

Pepper

Avocado

Radish

Cauliflower

Beet

Fennel

Jicama

Cabbage

Tomatillo

Lettuce

Broccoli

Sprout
Varieties

Varieties

Varieties

Bamboo
Shoots

Artichoke

Taro

Rutabaga

Kolhrabi

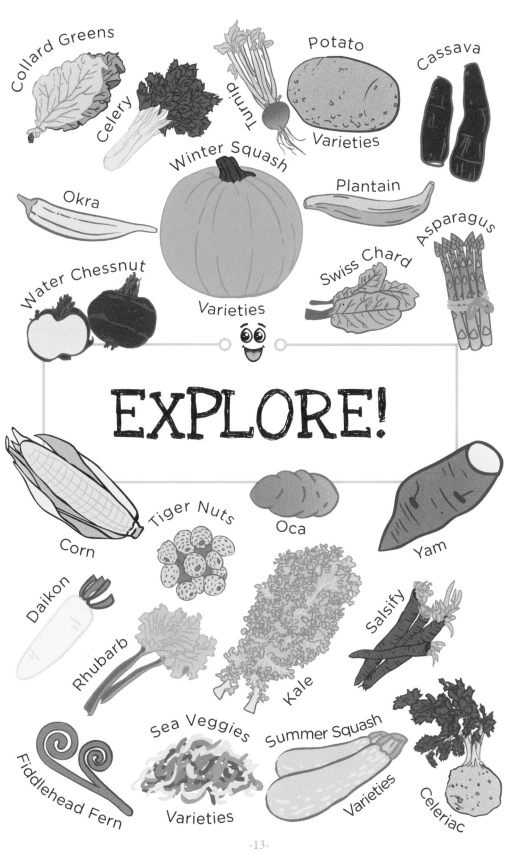

Collard Greens
Celery
Turnip
Potato Varieties
Cassava
Okra
Winter Squash Varieties
Plantain
Water Chessnut
Swiss Chard
Asparagus

EXPLORE!

Corn
Tiger Nuts
Oca
Yam
Daikon
Rhubarb
Kale
Salsify
Fiddlehead Fern
Sea Veggies Varieties
Summer Squash Varieties
Celeriac

**Veggie Name** _____  **Date** _____

**Preparation Method** _____

## Did you like this veggie?

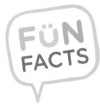

**FüN FACTS**

Lettuce varieties come in all different shapes, sizes, colors, and flavors. There are five common types of lettuce: butterhead, romaine, crisphead, leaf, and stem.

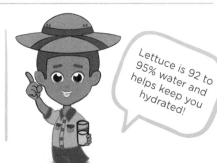

Lettuce is 92 to 95% water and helps keep you hydrated!

**Veggie Name** _____ **Date** _____

**Preparation Method** _____

## Did you like this veggie?

**Lettuce Varieties**

Arugula    Butterhead    Romaine    Crisphead    Endive    Leaf

**Veggie Name** _____ **Date** _____

**Preparation Method** _____

## Did you like this veggie?

## DID YOU KNOW?

A sip of water may taste sweet after eating an artichoke because of a natural acid that coats your mouth called cynarin. Try a bite of an artichoke and take a sip of water. Does it taste sweet?

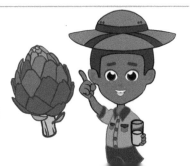

**Veggie Name** _____  **Date** _____

**Preparation Method** _____

_____

_____

_____

_____

_____

_____

_____

_____

_____

_____

## Did you like this veggie?

Draw
what
you're
tasting!

**Veggie Name** _____  **Date** _____

**Preparation Method** _____

_____
_____

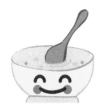
_____
_____

_____
_____

_____
_____

_____
_____

# Did you like this veggie?

**Cooking Method**

Soup and stew are preparation methods when liquids are boiled or simmered with ingredients such as meats, beans, and vegetables. Stews typically have less liquid than soups and are a thicker texture.

# Create your own vegetable soup!

**Draw your favorite veggies inside the pot and create a delicious soup!**

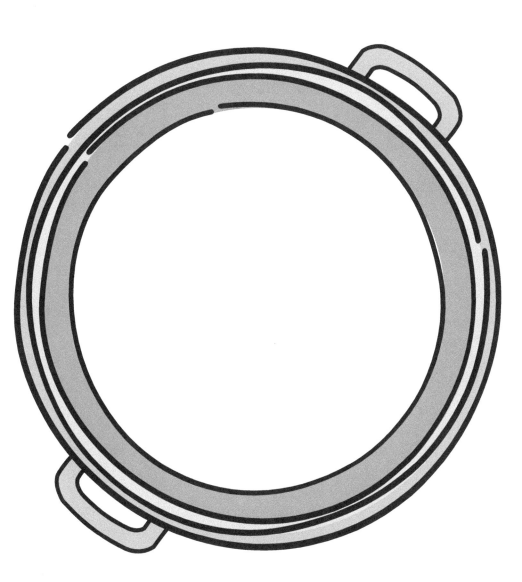

**Veggie Name** _____ **Date** _____

**Preparation Method** _____

## Did you like this veggie?

## DID YOU KNOW?

Temperature is a measurement that indicates how hot
or cold something is and can be measured using a
thermometer in degrees Fahrenheit or degrees Celsius.

**Veggie Name** _____ **Date** _____

**Preparation Method** _____

## Did you like this veggie?

### Tasting Notes

**Veggie Name** _____ **Date** _____

**Preparation Method** _____

## Did you like this veggie?

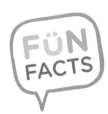

There are more than 200 varieties of potatoes sold throughout the United States. The differences in textures, flavors, and shapes make each variety unique.

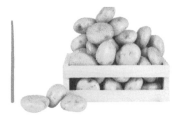

# Let's try
# Potato

Pick firm tubers. Avoid potatoes with green,
wrinkled skin, soft spots, cuts, and sprouts.

Color in this
Space-tator!

**Veggie Name** _____ **Date** _____

**Preparation Method** _____

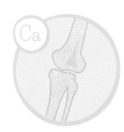

## Did you like this veggie?

### Good for My Body Nutrient

Calcium is a mineral that helps build strong bones and teeth, keeps your heart beating strong, and supports your body's nervous system.

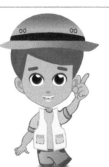

**Veggie Name** _____  **Date** _____

**Preparation Method** _____

_____

_____

_____

_____

_____

_____

_____

_____

_____

_____

# Did you like this veggie?

## DID YOU KNOW?

Have you ever heard the saying "cool as a cucumber?" The inside flesh of a cucumber growing in a field on a hot summer day is 20 degrees cooler than the outside air temperature!

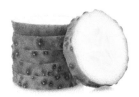

**Veggie Name** _____  **Date** _____

**Preparation Method** _____

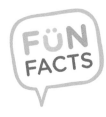

# Did you like this veggie?

**FÜN FACTS**

The terms Summer and Winter squash may be confusing because both types of squash grow during summer. Winter squash get their name from their thick, inedible skin that allows them to be stored and eaten several months after harvest.

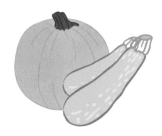

# Let's create a character with this pumkin!

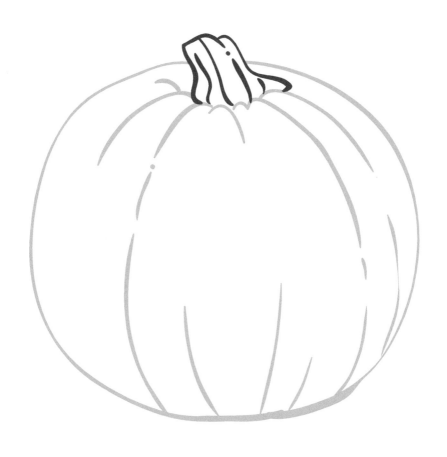

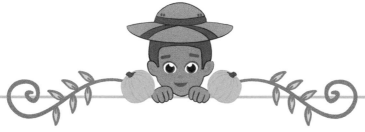

**Veggie Name** _____  **Date** _____

**Preparation Method** _____

# Did you like this veggie?

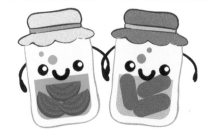

**Cooking Method**

Pickled or fermented foods are a preparation method that may include vinegar, brine, or helpful bacteria, also known as probiotics. Helpful bacteria support digestion and fight harmful bacteria.

**Veggie Name** ........................................................ **Date** ...................

**Preparation Method** ...................................................................

## Did you like this veggie?

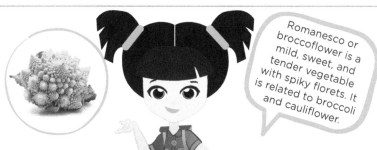

Romanesco or broccoflower is a mild, sweet, and tender vegetable with spiky florets. It is related to broccoli and cauliflower.

# Let's compare the same veggie prepared two ways!

**Veggie Name** _____ **Date** _____

**Preparation Method** _____

_____

_____

_____

_____

_____

_____

_____

_____

## Did you like this veggie?

**Which cooking method did you like better?**

_____

_____

**Veggie Name** _____ **Date** _____

**Preparation Method** _____

Did you like this veggie?

**Why did you like it?**

_____

_____

**Veggie Name** _____  **Date** _____

**Preparation Method** _____

## Did you like this veggie?

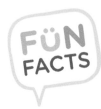

**FUN FACTS**

Corn is a fruit, vegetable, and grain! Corn is classified as a fruit because of how it grows; a vegetable when eaten fresh; and a grain when harvested as dry corn kernels.

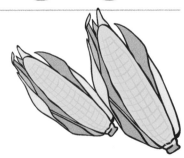

**Veggie Name** _____  **Date** _____

**Preparation Method** _____

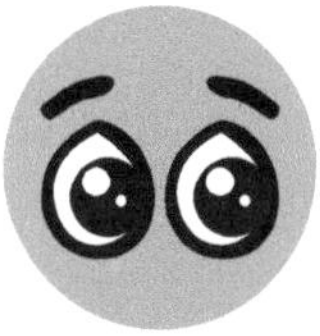

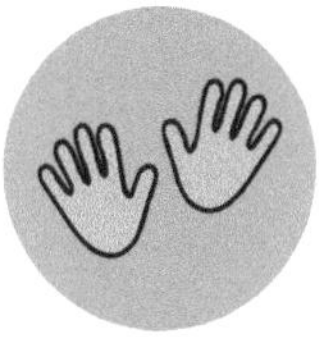

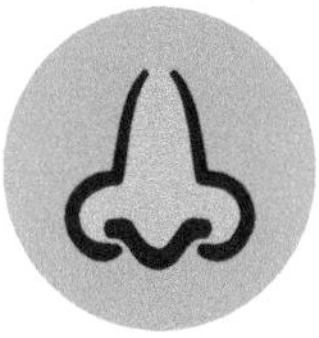

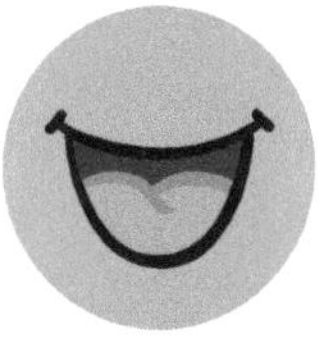

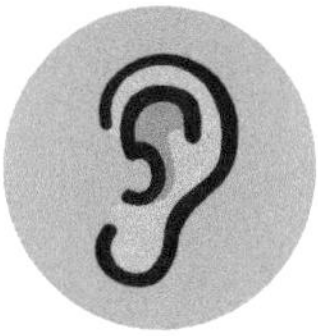

## Did you like this veggie?

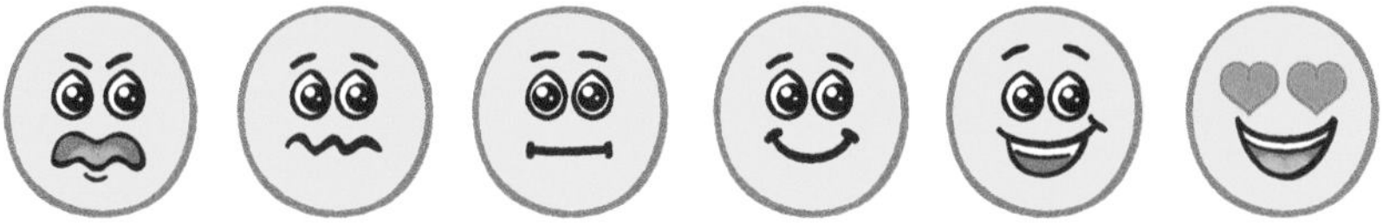

## Tasting Notes

_____

_____

_____

**Veggie Name** _____  **Date** _____

**Preparation Method** _____

## Did you like this veggie?

**FüN FACTS**

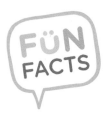

Peeled baby carrots are not actually baby carrots. They are fully grown carrots cut and shaped to a small size.

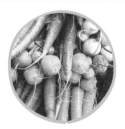

Carrots come in many different colors and shapes.

Why do you eat veggies?

How do you choose what
new veggies you will try?

**Veggie Name** _____ **Date** _____

**Preparation Method** _____

## Did you like this veggie?

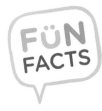

**FUN FACTS**

Chard is in the beet family but has been grown for its large, crisp leaves and multicolored stalks instead of its fleshy root. The flavor is described as a combination of beets and spinach.

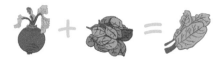

**Veggie Name** _____  **Date** _____

**Preparation Method** _____

_____

_____

_____

_____

_____

_____

_____

_____

_____

## Did you like this veggie?

Draw
what
you're
tasting!

**Veggie Name** _____  **Date** _____

**Preparation Method** _____

## Did you like this veggie?

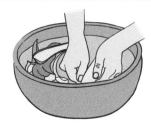

### DID YOU KNOW?

Green plantain skin may be peeled underwater to minimize bruising.

# Create a new veggie!
## Draw what it looks like and describe its flavors and textures.

**Veggie Name** _____ **Date** _____

**Preparation Method** _____

## Did you like this veggie?

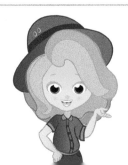 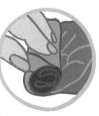 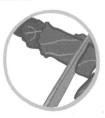

**CUTTING COLLARD GREENS**

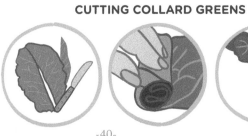

**Veggie Name** _____  **Date** _____

**Preparation Method** _____

# Did you like this veggie?

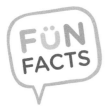

**Veggie Name** _____ **Date** _____

**Preparation Method** _____

## Did you like this veggie?

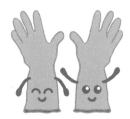

### DID YOU KNOW?

Yous should wear gloves to peel taro because it has oxalic acid in the raw flesh that may irritate the skin when peeled.

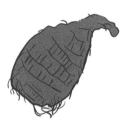

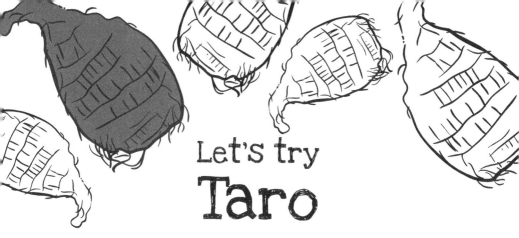

# Let's try
# Taro

Pick firm corms that are heavy for their size. Avoid taro with cuts, wrinkled skin, soft spots, and mold.

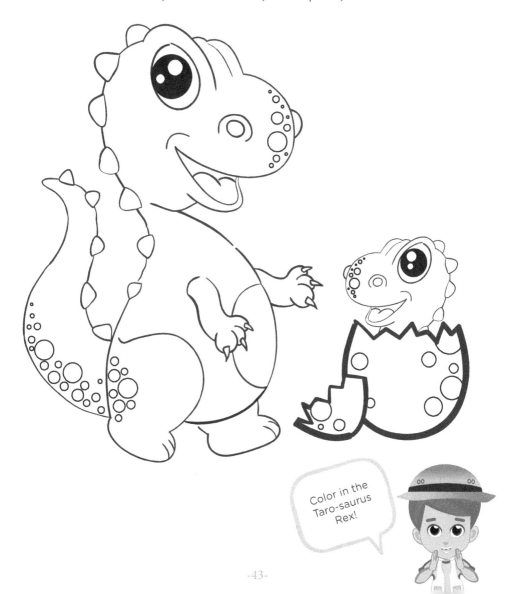

Color in the Taro-saurus Rex!

**Veggie Name** _____  **Date** _____

**Preparation Method** _____

## Did you like this veggie?

**FüN FACTS**

If you slice celery stems each piece makes the letter U!

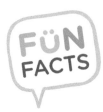

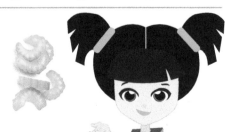

**Veggie Name**_____ **Date** _____

**Preparation Method** _____

## Did you like this veggie?

## Tasting Notes

# Let's compare the same veggie prepared two ways!

**Veggie Name** _____ **Date** _____

**Preparation Method** _____

## Did you like this veggie?

### Which cooking method did you like better?

_____

_____

# Let's compare the same veggie prepared two ways!

**Veggie Name** _____     **Date** _____

**Preparation Method** _____

## Did you like this veggie?

## Why did you like it?

_____

_____

**Veggie Name**_____ **Date** _____

**Preparation Method** _____

_____
_____

_____
_____

_____
_____

_____
_____

_____
_____

## Did you like this veggie?

Eggplant colors vary from deep purple or almost black, to light purple with creamy stripes, to all white. Eggplants also vary in shape from round, to pear-shaped, to long and cylindrical.

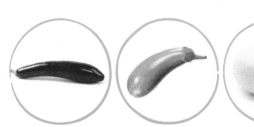

# Let's try veggie varieties!

**Veggie Name**

Draw the variety and describe its flavor using descriptive words.

**Variety:**

**Variety:**

**Variety:**

**Veggie Name**

Draw the variety and describe its flavor using descriptive words.

**Variety:**

**Variety:**

**Variety:**

**Veggie Name** _____  **Date** _____

**Preparation Method** _____

**Did you like this veggie?**

Veggies can grow above ground, below ground, or above and below ground. Other veggies flourish below water and some near water.

Above Ground | Below Ground | Above and Below Ground | Below or Near Water

**Veggie Name** _____ **Date** _____

**Preparation Method** _____

_____

_____

_____

_____

_____

_____

_____

_____

_____

_____

## Did you like this veggie?

Draw
what
you're
tasting!

**Veggie Name** _____ **Date** _____

**Preparation Method** _____

## Did you like this veggie?

## DID YOU KNOW?

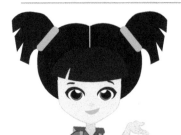

Okra is a natural thickening agent and can transform thin soups into thick broths and hearty stews. A delicious example of the thickening power of okra is gumbo.

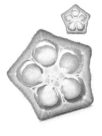

# Pick a veggie and draw what it looks like on the inside.

**Veggie Name** _____  **Date** _____

**Preparation Method** _____

## Did you like this veggie?

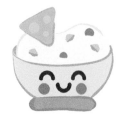

### Cooking Method

Dips, dressings, and sauces are foods prepared to be eaten as a topping or as an addition to other foods. They are available in many consistencies or textures from liquid, to semi-liquid, to thick, to chunky.

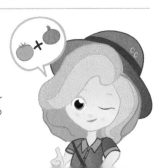

**Veggie Name** _____  **Date** _____

**Preparation Method** _____

_____

_____

_____

_____

_____

_____

_____

_____

_____

_____

_____

# Did you like this veggie?

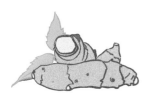

## DID YOU KNOW?

Jerusalem artichoke is a natural source of inulin, a type of fiber that cannot be digested by the body and may make you toot!

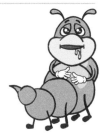

**Veggie Name** _____ **Date** _____

**Preparation Method** _____

## Did you like this veggie?

Wait to peel jicama skin until just before eating so the flesh doesn't dry out or harden.

**Veggie Name** _____ **Date** _____

**Preparation Method** _____

_____

_____

_____

_____

_____

_____

_____

_____

## Did you like this veggie?

Tasting Notes

_____

_____

**Veggie Name** _____  **Date** _____

**Preparation Method** _____

## Did you like this veggie?

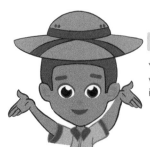

## DID YOU KNOW?

You can eat the entire plant for some veggies such as beets and carrots. This includes the root and leaves!

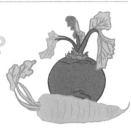

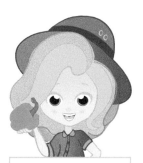

Baked     Boiled     Dessert     Dip

Garnish     Grill     Juice     Pickle

Raw     Sauté     Soup     Steam

**Tasting Notes**

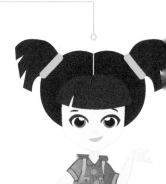

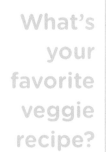

What's your favorite veggie recipe?

-59-

**Veggie Name** ........................................................ **Date** _____

**Preparation Method** _____

# Did you like this veggie?

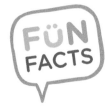

Slicing onions can make you cry! When you slice into an onion, a gas known as sulfoxide is released that stings your eyes. To keep eyes dry, chill onions in the refrigerator before chopping.

**Veggie Name** _____ **Date** _____

**Preparation Method** _____

# Did you like this veggie?

### Onion Varieties

Leek      Scallion      Shallot      Red Onion      White Onion      Yellow Onion

**Veggie Name** _____ **Date** _____

**Preparation Method** _____

## Did you like this veggie?

## Tasting Notes

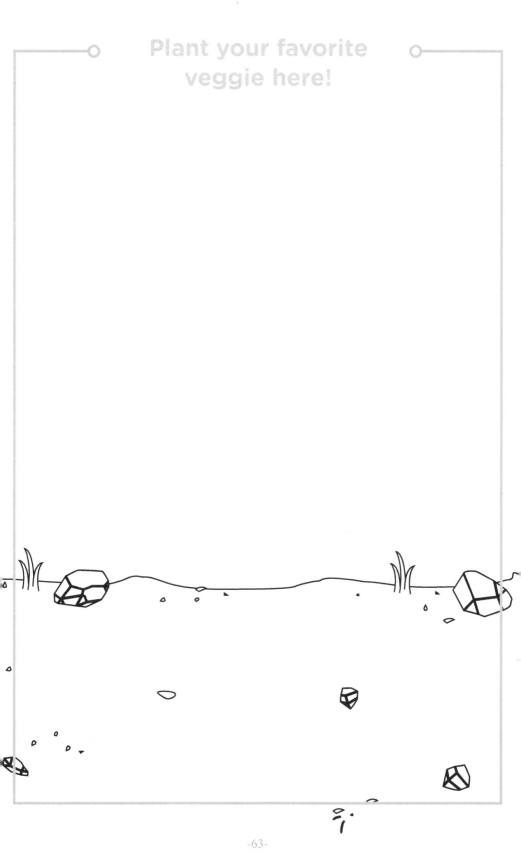

# Plant your favorite veggie here!

**Veggie Name** _____ **Date** _____

**Preparation Method** _____

## Did you like this veggie?

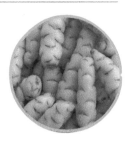

### DID YOU KNOW?

Oca are small and often about the size of a thumb. Varieties are pink-orange, yellow, apricot, and golden. The sun sweetens this tuber.

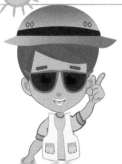

**Veggie Name** _____ **Date** _____

**Preparation Method** _____

_____

_____

_____

_____

_____

_____

_____

_____

_____

## Did you like this veggie?

Draw
what
you're
tasting!

**Veggie Name** _____ **Date** _____

**Preparation Method** _____

## Did you like this veggie?

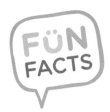

Daikon radishes can weigh up to 50 pounds!

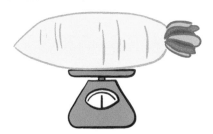

# Let's try
# Daikon

Pick white, firm, well-shaped roots with smooth skin. Avoid daikon with deep ridges and cuts. Attached greens should be bright green and crisp.

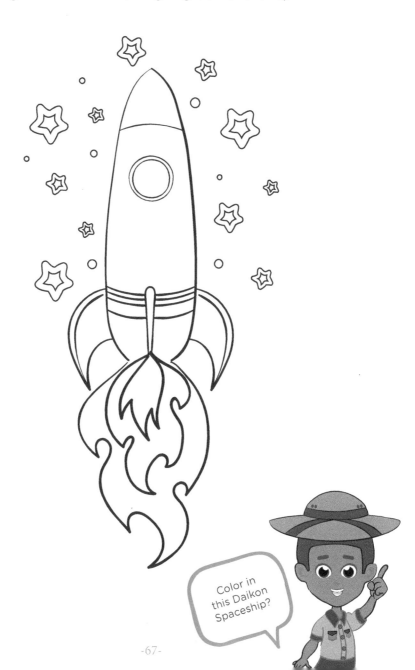

Color in this Daikon Spaceship?

**Veggie Name** _____ **Date** _____

**Preparation Method** _____

## Did you like this veggie?

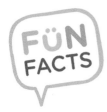

Green bell peppers left on the vine change color and become orange, red, and yellow. Extra time on the vine allows them to ripen which makes them sweeter.

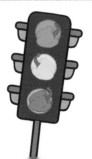

**Veggie Name** _____  **Date** _____

**Preparation Method** _____

## Did you like this veggie?

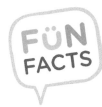

Seaweed is a name for plants and algae grown in marine or sea environments. There are three basic types of seaweed: brown, green, and red. The color depends on how close the seaweed grows to the surface of the ocean and the amount of sunlight it receives.

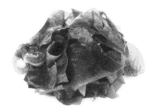

**Veggie Name** _____  **Date** _____

**Preparation Method** _____

## Did you like this veggie?

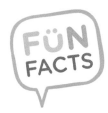

**FUN FACTS**

Scientists believe the fossils of the organism Prototaxites that date back more than 420 million years are giant fungus or mushrooms. This means mushrooms were around before dinosaurs roamed the earth!

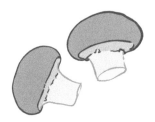

# Let's try veggie varieties!

## Veggie Name

Draw the variety and describe its flavor using descriptive words.

**Variety:**

**Variety:**

**Variety:**

## Veggie Name

Draw the variety and describe its flavor using descriptive words.

**Variety:**

**Variety:**

**Variety:**

**Veggie Name** _____  **Date** _____

**Preparation Method** _____

## Did you like this veggie?

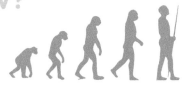

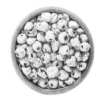

**Veggie Name** _____ **Date** _____

**Preparation Method** _____

_____

_____

_____

_____

_____

## Did you like this veggie?

Draw
what
you're
tasting!

**Veggie Name** _____ **Date** _____

**Preparation Method** _____

## Did you like this veggie?

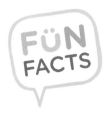

**FüN FACTS**

Fennel seeds are used for flavoring candy and foods such as pastries, pickles, and fish. It is also used in soaps and perfumes!

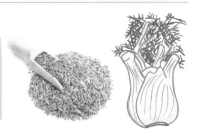

# Open your fridge and draw the veggies you see!

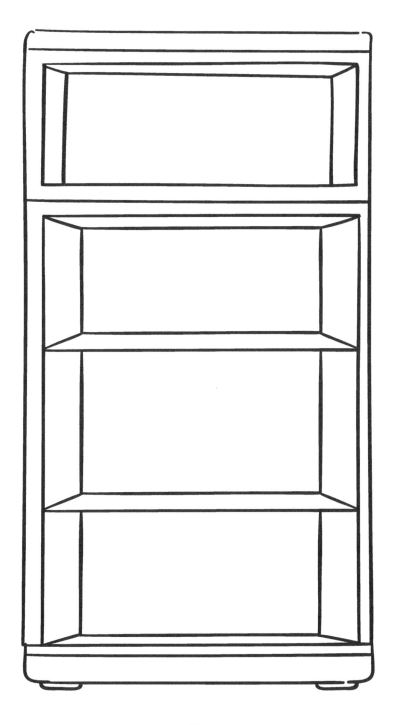

**Veggie Name**_____ **Date** _____

**Preparation Method** _____

_____

_____

_____

_____

_____

_____

_____

_____

_____

## Did you like this veggie?

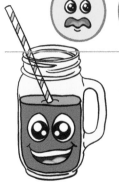

## DID YOU KNOW?

Spinach is the perfect addition to smoothies! It has a very mild flavor that is masked by fruit and a delicate texture that easily liquifies when blended.

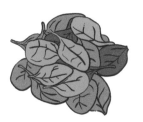

**Veggie Name** _____ **Date** _____

**Preparation Method** _____

## Did you like this veggie?

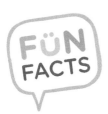

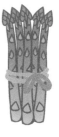

**Veggie Name** _____ **Date** _____

**Preparation Method** _____

# Did you like this veggie?

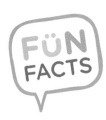

**FUN FACTS**

Most tomatoes found at grocery stores are picked and shipped green. They are artificially ripened with ethylene so they are red by the time you buy them. To keep your tomatoes plump and juicy, store them at room temperature on a flat surface with the stem side down.

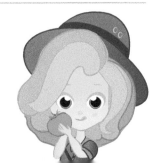

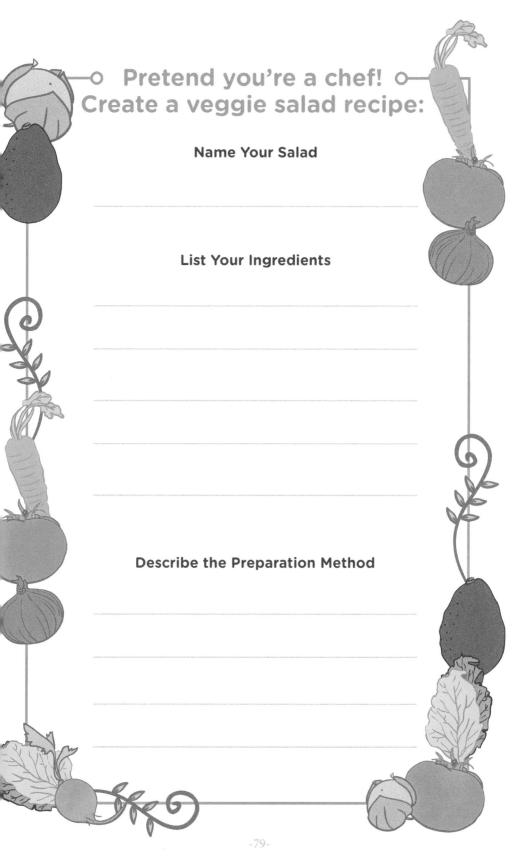

# Pretend you're a chef!
# Create a veggie salad recipe:

**Name Your Salad**

_____

**List Your Ingredients**

_____

_____

_____

_____

_____

**Describe the Preparation Method**

_____

_____

_____

_____

**Veggie Name** _____ **Date** _____

**Preparation Method** _____

_____

_____

_____

_____

_____

_____

_____

_____

_____

_____

## Did you like this veggie?

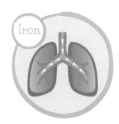

### Good for My Body Nutrient

Iron is a mineral that works like a big yellow school bus. It transports oxygen from your lungs to your whole body and keeps you moving.

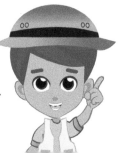

**Veggie Name** _____  **Date** _____

**Preparation Method** _____

## Did you like this veggie?

## Tasting Notes

**Veggie Name** _____  **Date** _____

**Preparation Method** _____

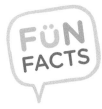

# Did you like this veggie?

**FüN FACTS**

Watercress is an aquatic or semi-aquatic leafy green related to the cabbage. It is considered a "Powerhouse Fruit and Vegetable" because it is an extremely nutrient dense green. This means it has a lot of Good For My Body Nutrients compared to the energy food will produce in your body.

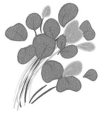

**Veggie Name** _____ **Date** _____

**Preparation Method** _____

## Did you like this veggie?

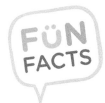

While the names are often used interchangeably, yams and sweet potatoes are not even the same type of vegetable. Yams are tubers and sweet potatoes are roots.

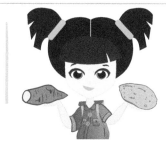

**Veggie Name** _____ **Date** _____

**Preparation Method** _____

## Did you like this veggie?

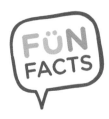

Water chestnuts are an aquatic vegetable. This means they grow by floating on the surface of water such as marshes, ponds, and lakes.

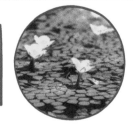

# Let's try veggie varieties!

**Veggie Name**

Draw the variety and describe its flavor using descriptive words.

**Variety:**

**Variety:**

**Variety:**

**Veggie Name**

Draw the variety and describe its flavor using descriptive words.

**Variety:**

**Variety:**

**Variety:**

## What did you discover by using this veggie journal?

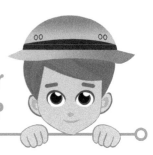

## How did you decide whether or not you liked a veggie?

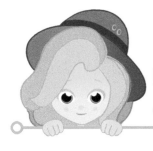

# Are there any textures you loved or disliked?

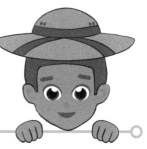

Crunchy · Fuzzy · Grainy · Meaty · Rubbery · Spongy · Tough

Continue your adventures in veggies and print additional "My 5 Senses Worksheets" from the Freebies tab on our website (www.experiencedeliciousnow.com)

Printed in the USA
CPSIA information can be obtained
at www.ICGtesting.com
LVHW071735210424
778001LV00035B/1615